ISBN: 978-0-557-25452-1

http://www.iwynn.net

iwynn is a registered trademark ® of iwynn productions and Isra Girgrah Wynn.

Editor: Michaela Brown
Layout and Cover Design: GMG World Media, LLC
Cover Photography: Roy Cox Photography
Isra Girgrah Wynn vs Christy Martin – August 23, 1997 / Photography: Teddy Blackburn

Acknowledgements:
Thanks to everyone who supports me in my vision to enlighten the world on wellness as a whole. I want to say a special thanks to my husband Marty Wynn for being there for me through everything and encouraging me to follow my dreams. I also want to thank my family for their guidance and for putting up with my non-traditional ways. Love you all.

This is dedicated to my grandmother "Gida" who died from Alzheimer's Disease before I could use this great information to help her live a little longer.

Table of Contents

Introduction

My name is Isra Girgrah Wynn. I am a retired, 5-time world champion, female professional boxer. I have been an athlete for most of my life and I enjoy the challenges of sports. After attending Queen's University in Canada, I took sports to the next level and competed professionally for 10 years. Nutrition has always been factor in my life because I was concerned with making weight. This, however, was not as important as being in the best physical shape to compete in the dangerous sport of boxing, or so I thought! What I gave my body for fuel, as the years went by, became much more important. I began to understand that the nutrients which drove my body to optimum health and fitness were more important than me being physically fit! I would always be just that...physically fit and have the skills to perform at competition level! The question I had to ask myself then was, "Is what I eat nutritionally sound for my performance?" What a revelation! This made me realize that I could have the best skills in the world, but if I wasn't eating the proper food to give me energy, fuel, and stamina, then the physical stuff didn't matter! WOW! I get it! This made life a whole lot easier especially when it came to competing. I was able to maximize on the knowledge of optimal health for peak performance! No one else knew that, and I believed I had the upper hand.

I have been involved in health, nutrition, and fitness for the majority of my life. In the beginning, I only concentrated on the fitness aspect of health. As the years passed, I became more aware of the importance of nutrition and therefore, continued to further my education with classes at different institutes. Everyone gets minimal exercise during the day, but it's done unconsciously. Pushing and pulling doors, walking up and down stairs, and sitting and getting up from chairs, are all forms of exercise. Fitness and strength are not synonymous with health! Jogging and other strenuous exercise should never be used to "get healthy." Health begins in the kitchen. Your meals should be healthy. Then, you can exercise to tone muscle and maintain strength.

What we consume for fuel tremendously lacks nutritional value. This is why I started studying health and wellness from a nutritional stand point. I discovered a long time ago that being healthy is key to maintaining a great, disease- and pain-free life. It allows me to do things that I wouldn't be able to do if I were not conscious of what I eat and how I treat my body. I'm human like everyone else. I am not perfect and I have cravings. I eat what I want, on occasion, but I do it rarely. Temptations are everywhere. You have to be conscious of what you eat, drink and think. I want to help the general public become more aware about nutrition, optimum health, and wellness. Things that you want to know, but don't want to read a whole book about, are covered in this book. This book includes simplified tips you can take with you on your everyday trek.

Our first reaction to an illness is to either self-medicate, with over-the-counter medications, or go to the doctor's office and he or she might prescribe you medication. Have you ever asked your doctor if there is an alternative way to treat the illness? Most likely, you haven't or you never thought to ask because the doctor is a "professional." Unfortunately, the medications we take may cause other problems which may develop later in life when the actual problem has accelerated to a bigger issue. Medications are prescribed to relieve symptoms. Unfortunately , the problem that causes the symptoms still exist. Medications are not designed to cure the diseases of the body, they are prescribed to soothe and make the disease less serious. Treating symptoms will not correct the cause. My point is, people should continue to educate themselves and take life, and health, more seriously. We only have one. Why not enjoy it the right way! I am not a doctor. I am not telling anyone not to see a doctor or not to take medications. I am merely saying that people need to eat better, and over time, the body will correct itself. See if you can live illness free or even lessen the severity of these problems. Taking the steps to make a conscious decision to live life to the fullest will be rewarding!

Let's get started with these small tips that people should know. You, and only YOU, are responsible for your own health. Health is more than the absence of pain. "Making small changes makes a big difference!! Life is short, make the most of it!"

I am writing this book with the hopes that it gives

you, the reader, awareness about the importance of health and nutrition for wellness. When we were born, we were perfect until we started ingesting food and living in poor environments. We have veered off the path. We need to get back on track with more nutritious food choices. The average individual is not aware that little things can make a difference. The tips in this book can be used as a guide to make better choices and begin living a much healthier lifestyle. Lifestyle is the primary determinant of health. Nutrition doesn't stand alone in the path to good health and wellness. We all need exercise, fresh air, sunshine, adequate rest, recreation, and sufficient self discipline to stop and smell the roses now and then.[1] I hope this proves helpful to you. All of the information in this book has been researched or has been found through personal experience, over the years. Please consult with you doctor or a physician before changing your diet or lifestyle.

"Why don't we make health and
nutrition priorities in our lives?"

Chapter 1
Thought Process

"Let your food be your medicine!!" The kitchen is more important to our health than the doctor's office or the local hospital![2] It has always been a mystery to me why people don't take their health seriously enough to make small changes in their lives. We complain about the little things in life, but these little things are because of our health. Most people who have a life threatening illness are eager to try anything that might give them a glimmer of hope to improving their circumstances. Those who suffer pain or chronic discomforts are generally motivated to try just about anything to relieve their symptoms. Why does it take extreme circumstances to get people to leave their comfort zone? Being a little uncomfortable will sometimes go a long way! No one wants to sacrifice the rich, sweet tastes for a better way of living. The good news is we don't have to give them up completely. The transition to a more advantageous way of eating for a lifetime of good health doesn't have to be overwhelming or traumatic! A few small changes will begin to make a difference.

The mind is powerful! If you put your mind to something, you can achieve it!! The mind is so powerful it can actually manifest disease. Usually when I am stressed, I don't feel good, however, when I am happy, I feel great! This is done through negative thoughts and stress, which we will talk about later. It's like a double-edged sword. Great nutrition is needed for proper brain function. You want to be able to think clearer, faster, and more precise, without fog or distractions. Your IQ today could be the result of the nutrition consumed by your ancestors while they were pregnant, traced down to your mother and how she ate while pregnant with you. A fetus is very sensitive to the nutrients it receives while in the womb. Getting the right ones are essential for the proper growth of an unborn child. There are critical periods of growth during the 9-10 months of fetal development, as well as the first few years of life. It is the mother's duty to provide the best nutrients to her fetus for optimum growth. This sets the standard for each person as they grow to become independent and eventually make their own choices in life. Any substance that interferes with the natural workings of the body is a toxin, food included.

I have studied that most of our illnesses may be linked to improper diets. Diet in this sense means the way an individual eats daily, not these "fad" diets that claim to make you skinny or lose weight quickly! We are not eating well-balanced meals throughout the day. The nutrients we should get from our meals are insufficient in every form. We have settled for the fast or quick-and-easy meals, constantly compromising our health!

There are 50 essential nutrients needed for optimum health.[3] Let's break down what they are – two fats, nine amino acids (from protein), 21 minerals, 13 vitamins, plus carbohydrates, fiber, light, oxygen, and water. There are other non-essential nutrients, as well. These non-essential nutrients are made by the body naturally.

Our food preferences, desires, cravings, and loves are controlled from the center of our brain. What you eat directly and indirectly affects chemicals which, in turn, influence your mood, energy level, food craving, stress level and sleep habits. If your diet doesn't include enough vitamins and minerals, your mood appetite, and thinking are also affected. We will talk about how this happens in a later chapter.

There's a host of other environmental issues which also contributes to our bodies not getting proper nutrients. If you are able to consume the recommended daily allowance of nutrients, your entire body, including your skeleton, will begin to gradually rebuild over time. You can choose to nourish your body or you can choose to abuse your body. You are the one who decides how you live, what you eat, and what you think. With optimum nutrition, you can possibly increase your IQ, physical performance, improve mental clarity, mood, concentration, quality of sleep, resistance to infections, protect yourself from disease, and extend your healthy life span. That's a lot! It has been proven through research.[4]

"The evidence for nutritional therapy is becoming so strong that if the doctors of today don't become nutritionists, the nutritionists will become the doctors of tomorrow!!"[5] This is where our society is headed, so why not begin making changes now before it is too late! Some essential nutrients activate the body's processes to perform certain functions. Vitamins "turn on" enzymes (discussed later), which, in turn, make body processes happen. Minerals are also necessary for proper body function. They play many key roles in human health. The nutrients we get from the food we eat (fuel, or energy as we often say) are what drive our bodies (like premium gas in a car) to optimum health and ultimate wellness. We would be healthier if we took heed to a few tips that could change our lives forever. We could possibly add a few more years of great, pain-free living to our lives so we can enjoy it with our family and friends. The doctors and pharmaceutical companies wouldn't be happy...but we would!

Chapter 2
Body – Healthy or Diseased

Food is fuel for the body. It oxidizes during digestion to produce energy. Food produces internal energy to
maintain a constant temperature and keep your organs and
systems functioning.[6] "Unless we put foods in our bodies
that have the right chemical balance needed to sustain good
health, we are hopelessly unable to resist disease."[7]

Disease and poor health are not accidental. Health
is defined as the normal, optimum performance of the body
and mind.[8] Disease is an imbalance or disturbance in function.[9] It is the inability of the body to maintain a consis-
tently normal environment, internally. When you violate
nature's laws, you compromise your health and develop
disease. You can eat, drink, and think yourself into disease.
So, if you want a natural way to slow or reverse the effects of disease, you MUST change your eating habits. The
development of a disease is a slow process, beginning with
small changes in your body. If these changes aren't cor-
rected through proper nutrition, the body will compensate,
internally, to correct itself. Once the body starts compensat-
ing, it produces symptoms. And, if this continues without
positive changes, it can cause physical signs of disease.

The brain controls every part of your body. If this control center is not working properly, then nothing else will. Impaired mental function always comes before physical problems. Look at your diet also before blaming your age or heredity factors for lapses in memory, thinking, or concentration. You must take every avenue into consideration when trying to find solutions to these physical and mental issues. People who eat a good breakfast think better and faster, remember more, react quicker, and are mentally sharper than breakfast skippers.[10] The brain is fuel fussy, demanding that all its energy come from glucose (the fuel from sweets and starchy foods). Make sure you make the right choice though! The body is intelligent. Everything that happens inside the body is caused by something. The body works only for immediate survival, not towards long-term health and happiness. We have a built in survival instinct which handles threats. You may not be consciously aware that your body is responding to past events. But, in time, you may begin to experience pain and illness because your body is stressed.

Everyone wants to be in great physical health, regardless of age. Age is not an excuse for disease. Older people may become ill and develop diseases due to long-term neglect of their health, which affects them later in life. For years, they live with issues of poor nutrition and their bodies must work overtime to maintain stability as long as possible. There is a genetic and hereditary factor to take into consideration as well. Making better choices helps in the long run.

When your body is really healthy, i.e., performing at

optimum levels, bad bacteria can't penetrate your immune defenses. You have to understand how your body works in order to stay healthy. Body chemistry teaches you how and why you need certain amounts of nutrients. You also have to understand how food works for your body. Food chemistry teaches you the best food sources for those essential nutrients. Every body function is a response to a stimulus— food stress, thoughts, lifestyle. Pain or discomfort caused by the response is called a symptom. These "symptoms" are signals that your body is adapting to survive the stimulus. Your body doesn't know how to be sick. Symptoms are signs that you have pushed your body's natural healing systems beyond their limits. Committing to better health and wellness is personal and specific to each individual. All I can do is provide you with information to help you make it easier. It starts with you. Make a decision to achieve a goal and stick to this commitment until the end.

Chapter 3
Our Ingenious Body

Let's begin with a few things about the human body which will provide you with a clear picture of what we are dealing with. Nothing created by man compares to the design of the human body. The body has an unexplainable and awesome internal intelligence. A higher being created us with the intentions of our bodies taking care of themselves without our knowing. The body knows exactly what to do in order to survive as long as possible. Everything that happens inside your body is caused by something. Again, symptoms are signals of the body adapting to survive the things to which it is exposed. These warnings signs are your body's way of telling you that its natural health potential has been compromised.

The body provides clues for us to correct the problem. For example, fevers and colds are the body's survival tactics. A fever kills off intruders so the body can resume its regular routine. This is one way the body flushes toxins. A cold's purpose is another way for the body to rid itself of toxins which threaten its survival. You just don't catch a cold or come down with a fever. They are natural, periodic cleansing functions by the body to eliminate accumulated toxins. Therefore, they are beneficial and necessary.

The body has a series of integrated systems, each having a specific role or task. These roles are complicated and they all work simultaneously. There are eleven body systems. They are skeletal, muscular, nervous, skin/hair/nails, lymphatic/immune, endocrine, cardiovascular, respiratory, digestive, urinary, and reproductive. These intricate systems work together to maintain health and efficiency. Unlike a new car, we come without a maintenance manual or warranty. Most of us think about body maintenance only when something goes wrong. Most illnesses and complications take a long time to develop. When we finally notice the symptoms, it may be too late. Some diseases take twenty to thirty years to develop. Why? The body is a highly sophisticated machine. It tries to fix itself, by compromising other parts, before it lets us know something is wrong. Even though our body might warn us about a problem, it will develop symptoms from the last problem that occurred or the last part that was compromised in the process of fixing the first one!

It's easy to mistake the symptom for the problem. Here's an example. In the condition known as osteoporosis (softening of the bone), mineral levels remain normal in the blood while the body gradually removes minerals from the bones, due to a calcium deficiency in our nutrient intake. It's like robbing Peter to pay Paul! The body constantly compensates for our nutritional mistakes. With vitamin and mineral deficiencies, the body is forced to take nutrients from other systems because they are urgently needed to supplement an even more crucial job! These are the intricate details of the human body which make it complicated and brilliant! We know these conditions as diseases but with more balance in nutrition, we might be able to reduce the severity of these problems. Does that make sense?

Many people believe that when they get sick, there's an easy fix…like we can just take medication to solve the problem. What is the actual problem? Why are doctors prescribing medication? Doctors prescribe these medications for the symptoms, not the problems or the cause. How many doctors are going to ask you what you ate over the last 2-3 months or if you have been taking vitamin and mineral supplements? Would they ask you how much water you've consumed over the last few months? NO! They studied to determine treatment for specific symptoms and to prescribe medication for them. Then, a few months later, you return to their office for more medicine because the previous medicine caused side effects which made your body go haywire! Taking any drug –prescription, over-the-counter, or street – introduces chemicals into the body that it was never designed to process. Your organs hold on to chemicals from medications for years! Often, toxic substances are stored in body fat, genetically weak organs and tissues, and the bones. They don't completely flush out of your system, but there are ways to start developing a healthier body. As I said earlier, I am not a doctor. I am not telling you not to take medications, nor am I telling you not see a doctor. Just research other avenues to reduce the effects of illnesses.

Chapter 4
Water-Fluid

The human body possesses a variety of sophisticated indicators when it runs short of water. These emergency indicators are dehydration and thirst.[11] The human body is approximately composed of 60-75% water.[12] This percentage varies by individual. The brain is approximately 75% water; muscles are almost 75% water; the lungs are approximately 86% water; the heart is approximately 75% water; the liver is approxiamtely 96% water; the blood is approximately 83% water; even approximately 20% of bone is water.[13] That's a lot of water! Water helps regulate the body's acidity and body temperature. If you don't drink enough water to replenish the body's natural loss, its systems will suffer.

The recommended intake of water is eight cups, or 64 ounces, every day! How is this number computed? Well it is said that you lose ten glasses, equaling approximately 80 ounces, of water every day![14] How is this number calculated? Here's the breakdown: two glasses from evaporating and sweating, two glasses from breathing, and six glasses through waste removal.[15] We replace two glasses through the food and fluids we consume but we still need 8 more glasses![16] If you exercise, you have to add more water to your intake! So now you are looking at consuming approximately 9-13 glasses daily. That's a lot of water to drink!!! You can get it from a variety of sources including, plain water, juices, tea, etc.

"Fluids" and "water" are not necessarily the same. The mistaken assumption that all fluids are equal to water for the water needs of our bodies might be the main cause of many of the problems and illnesses. I have experienced this first hand. Trying to drink anything other that water, because of taste, I ended up not getting what I needed and also ended up eating more! Be aware that caffeine-containing beverages act as a diuretic (increased urine production) and causes water loss. These beverages, like soda, in excess, may cause dehydration. They might also create a slight increase in weight, from overeating as a direct result of confusion between thirst and hunger sensations. I will explain on the next page. Even though you might think you are doing something right, in reality, you are still losing water! Be aware of this point. Diet sodas contain artificial sweeteners, which are approximately 180 times sweeter than sugar without any calories. These beverages also cause hunger, masking the thought of satisfying your thirst. We tend to eat more because of the thirst/hunger sensation that is often confusing.

Your urine is an important indicator of how much water you need. If it is dark in color, you are not drinking enough water. If it is light, you are drinking enough. This is not the only way to gauge it. Taking supplements, like a multi-vitamin with B-complex vitamins or B vitamins (especially B12), gives the urine a florescent yellow hue, much different from dark yellow. Just make a conscious effort to drink a glass of water every 1-2 hours. This helped me control my water intake. Another indication of dehydration is thirst. This is a sign that you are already slightly dehydrated! The simple truth is that dehydration may cause disease at severe levels.[17] Thirst is a symptom of dehydration. When you have lost between 1-2% of body water, the thirst mechanism is activated. Make sure you don't mistake it for hunger.

The sensation of thirst and hunger are generated at the same time. We do not recognize the difference. We eat when we are thirsty but instead, the body should receive water, hence the statement made on the previous page referencing weight gain. How I can tell the difference is by drinking two glasses of water before I eat. After about 20 minutes, if I am still hungry, then I eat. If not, then it was my body's way of telling me that it is mildly dehydrated. You can separate the two sensations by doing this. If you are constantly thirsty and you drink lots of fluids, it could be from blood sugar problems (blood sugar levels are too high; diabetics) or you are deficient in essential fat (not consuming enough good fat; e.g. fish, seeds, nuts).[18] Consult with your doctor or physician at this point to make sure. Mild dehydration can lead to headaches, constipation, lethargy, and mental confusion. It can also put you at risk of recurring urinary tract infections and kidney stones. Kidney stones also form from too much protein caused by the build-up of uric acid.[19]

When three percent of your body water is lost, it

seriously affects mental and physical performance. In athletes, an eight percent of muscle strength is lost when this happens! I have seen this happen many times in the sport I participated. Boxing requires you to lose weight to get to a designated class. Most boxers do not do this the healthy way. They end up losing a considerable amount of water weight a few weeks before the event to make that weight. This ends up being extremely dangerous to ones health as they enter the ring and participate in this barbaric sport. I learned this early in my career, and I tried to stay a pound or two within fight weight, for the most part.

Not drinking enough water can cause other health problems, such as gastric ulcers, joint pain, asthma and allergies. "Dry mouth" is the very last sign of dehydration. Be careful, though. On the other side, you can also drink too much water. Drinking too much water taxes the kidneys and can cause over hydration. If taken to an extreme, it can kill you. These cases are rare but are still possible. Make sure you drink the right amount of water and consult with a physician!

Chapter 5
Breakdown of Food & Combining Foods

We are what we eat! Sound familiar? We hear it often. What does that really mean? Let me rephrase that. We are what we can digest and absorb! Nutrients drive us. They are the fuel which allows us to live on a daily basis. The type of fuel we consume and how we internally process it determine how well our bodies run! It's like putting sugar in the gas tank of a car! Not a smart idea because the car will definitely not run! So the question becomes, "would you put anything other than premium fuel into a Bentley or a Rolls Royce?". NO! We need to treat our bodies like shrines or like we treat our luxury cars!! Why do we put so much sugar into our bodies? IT JUST TASTES GREAT! Yes, Lord, it does! Fat and sugar taste great! However, there are many consequences and repercussions from consuming it. We will explain to you how fat and sugar taste great later.

When we consume food and beverages high in sugar, it's almost like we are on a high! And, honestly, we are! The effects of sugar and/or carbohydrates are almost like a drug. We want more! Why? The body releases chemicals which make us want more. Our bodies make us think we are not satisfied after eating. In other words, we believe we are still hungry and we keep eating! Now this is great information, so pay attention! Within minutes of consuming carbohydrates, the body releases insulin, a powerful chemical hormone produced by the pancreas. The amount of insulin released depends on the amount of carbohydrates eaten in previous meals. Consuming large amounts of carbohydrates increases the level of insulin in the bloodstream.

Insulin helps deliver energy to the body's organs. As this happens, the insulin level in the bloodstream drops and causes the brain to release a chemical called serotonin. This is the brain's "happy chemical." Many people who have low levels of serotonin feel depressed and tend to eat more. Serotonin also controls appetite. The more serotonin the brain releases, the less you eat. The presence of serotonin produces a feeling of satisfaction. Insulin is sometimes called the hunger hormone because it stimulates the appetite. Insulin may cause a person to feel hungrier than they initially thought. The brain receives a signal to stop eating and the insulin level drops. The amount of insulin in the bloodstream changes hours later and the sensation of hunger returns. The cycle repeats if you continue eating carbohydrates and don't balance the meal with protein and good fats. If an excess of insulin remains in the bloodstream, serotonin fails to rise and a person will not feel satisfied.

Because we have become a "fast and right now" society, many processed food products are conveniently available to us. We are conditioned to consume more carbohydrates to satisfy our hunger, which repeats the cycle we mentioned earlier. We must learn how to properly balance our meals. When we consume white sugar, lots of energy is produced. Unfortunately, at the same time, the body produces high levels of acid. This process doesn't stimulate beneficial minerals to neutralize it, which may cause hyperactivity and hyper-irritability. The body is unable to efficiently process a flood of fast-releasing sugars. It sends your blood sugar levels through the roof! Once this flood is set in motion, other hormones swing into emergency action to restore balance and feeds potentially undesirable microorganisms that can occur in the gut! That's a lot for the body to handle.

A well-balanced meal consists of protein (meat, poultry, eggs, tofu, fish), carbohydrates (bread, pasta, potatoes, rice, sugar, fruits, vegetables), fats (nuts, oils, butter, margarine), and fiber. The ones you decide to eat, with consultation, are important as well. Another important aspect when choosing what to eat is the way we combine those foods. The process of determining food compatibility is important so digestion occurs smoothly. NO PUN INTENDED!! All we know how to do is put food into our body and the stomach has to sort through it. It takes different secretions and times to digest different foods. For example, it takes approxiamtely 15-20 minutes to digest fruit and sugar when eaten alone.[20] However, it takes approximately five hours for the body to digest meat.[21] This is recommended to be your last meal of the day. Protein digestion needs an acidic environment, while starch digestion needs and alkaline environment.[22]

It's not a good idea to combine meat and a sugary carbohydrate for dessert. The sugar becomes caught in the digestion of the meat! This makes the sugar ferment and produces gas! Sound familiar? I'm sure we have all experienced this at one time or another. Some more than others! HINT: when proteins are not fully digested, they generate gases and cause stomach rumblings, gas pains, and flatuous odor (from the bottom)! This is called putrefaction, or rotting! When carbohydrates are not properly digested, they ferment and cause gas and belching (from the top). Fats that are not oxidized or decomposed turn rancid. These unused materials are left behind after digestion. Where does all that unusable waste go?

The intestines of an average adult contain approximately 5-30 pounds of undigested fecal matter, that is, if you haven't gotten a colonic or had a body cleanse (detoxification)! The colon, on an average, is two inches in diameter. Poor eating habits and drugs can allow for accumulation of fecal matter to stretch the colon as large as five inches in diameter. A prime example of this was the examination of Elvis Presley's colon after his death. He loved the traditional meat and potatoes meal. (Urban Legends Reference Pages. (1995-2009). Barbara and David P. Mikkelson. Retrieved from http://www.snopes.com/horrors/gruesome/fecalcolon.asp) The undigested food gathers in your intestines. It forms toxins that are absorbed into the bloodstream. Toxins are poisonous to the body. They are in air, water, food, and other ingested substances. The more rotting or putrefaction that takes place, the more constipated the person becomes. This word, constipation, is misunderstood by the public. Constipation should be understood as not having at least one bowel movement a day! I have experienced a colonic or two in my time and it is shocking to see how much unusable food stays in the bowels. I try to incorporate fiber into my diet so that it can clean out my intestines and keep them safe and healthy from toxins. Another benefit that colonics presented to me was, it made me lose weight, depending on how clean I ate!!

Everyone should detoxify and rest their bodies from time to time. Consult your doctor before trying a detoxification program. The way we eat, the lifestyles we live, the illnesses we might have, and the way we eliminate waste all depend on how frequently we should detoxify. There is a wide selection of detoxification programs and it is nice to just give your body a break from all the unhealthy food we consume, as well as limiting our exposure to environmental influences.

So you see, it's important to properly combine food for easy digestion. Properly combining foods relieves the body of the sorting process. The stomach processes foods in order of dominance, whichever is more abundant in the food, carbohydrates, proteins, and/or fats. Then it moves to the next abundant constituent and so on. Enzymes that begin the breakdown of carbohydrates are released in the mouth and enzymes that begin the breakdown of proteins are released in the stomach (we will talk more about this later). The general rule of thumb when food combining is that vegetables can be eaten with any other food category. Fruit is recommended to be eaten alone. Starch, dairy and meat, generally, should not be eaten together. If you stick to this general rule of thumb, your system may digest better so you can get the most nutrients out of the food you eat. You'll possibly become more regular so there won't be much in your intestines. Since your system will work better, you'll be hungry more often. This, in turn, will speed up your metabolism and allow you to burn fat easier or maintain your weight. This will also allow you to have more energy! Sounds great doesn't it! When I found out about food combining and applied that concept to my life-style, I felt so much better. I was digesting better, using nu-trients more efficiently, and I felt hungrier every two hours because the food wasn't caught up in my stomach or intes-tines for hours. I was able to maintain my weight and even lose weight easier, which took the stress of weighing in off of me. This was valuable to me because of the demands of the sport I chose to be a part of.

Chapter 6
Energy-Stress-Nutrients

The body's two basic attributes are energy and nutri-ents. Glucose, the byproduct of carbohydrates when they are digested and converted, is fuel ignited by oxygen (in the air we breath and in the food we eat) to produce energy. Energy is the ability to do work. It is measured in calories and food is the fuel on which our body runs. You must make sure you are getting the right calories. Many foods, like sodas, sugary foods, and processed foods, have empty calo-ries. Lack of energy can be attributed to lack of nutrients, as well as stress.

Stress is one of the most common health problems associated with a variety of illnesses in the US.[23] Stress begins in the mind. Signals stimulate the adrenal glands to produce adrenaline as well as cortisol. Short bursts of cortisol are helpful for stress but long term exposure may be toxic to the brain and the body. Cortisol reduces the brain's ability to use glucose as well as affects the functioning of chemicals like serotonin. Some causes of stress may be emotions (anger, fear, worry, anxiety), excess sugar, insuf-ficient rest and sleep, or dietary and lifestyle stimulants (cigarettes, caffeine, pills). The adrenal glands sit on top of the kidneys and produce hormones that, among other things, help us adapt to stress. In seconds, your heart is pounding, your breathing changes, muscles tense, eyes dilate, blood thickens (to have the ability to help wounds heal) and stored glucose is released into the blood. Your body chemistry changes every time you react to a stressful situation. It could be as simple as a stressful thought. I can just imagine what my body chemistry looked like on the inside when I was preparing for a fight! Probably havoc!! I endured stress leading up to a fight, not only physical stress but also emotional. I had to incorporate a lot of exercises in anti-stress like, breathing, mental imagery, and positive affirmations.

Thoughts exert the most powerful influence on your health and negative thoughts are the number one acid producers in the body.[24] When in a defensive state (even from past conditions that no longer exist), the body produces more acid than it can process. Your body responds to negative mental and emotional stress brought about by thoughts in exactly the same way it reacts to real threats of physical harm! Physiologists have found that thoughts are so influential, all you have to do is anticipate exercise for the nervous system to stimulate cardiac output![25] Can we THINK ourselves into shape? Good question! That's HUGE!!

Consequences from the adrenal glands becoming exhausted may be immune system failure, irregular sleep patterns, weight loss, bone loss, fat accumulation around the waist, increased blood sugar, and elevated blood fat levels. Conservative estimates suggest you double your need for vitamins when you are in a stressed state.[26] The extra energy associated with being stressed results from your body's normal repair and maintenance jobs like digestion, cleansing, etc. The energy is redirected from these processes to combat stress. People also turn to food to soothe their feelings. Anxiety, worries, tension, upset feelings, stress, and fear are common causes of emotional eating. Food ends up being the solution to helping you through tough times. I know I have definitely experienced that!! Cheese cake solved all my problems at times of stress and PMS! Oops! We live and learn.

When energy levels drop, we turn to stimulants like coffee, sugar, tea, chocolate, sodas, cigarettes, and other legal and illegal stimulants. These stimulants cause the release of adrenalin, but it has a negative effect. The body slows digestion, repair, and maintenance to deal with it. The cycle causes dependency (addiction) on the stimulants. These stimulants aren't helpful and are unhealthy. By living off stimulants such as coffee, cigarettes, high-sugar foods, or stress itself, you increase your risk of upsetting your thyroid balance or calcium balance. Your metabolism will slow down, you will gain weight, and could possibly develop arthritis. These are the long-term side effects of stress. Any body system that is overstimulated will eventually under-function. Reduce your stress level by reducing your intake of sugar and stimulants.

Every muscle cell you hold in tension consumes energy! It has been happening for decades and even happens while you sleep. You must find ways to relax!! Take up a sport, get a monthly or weekly massage, meditate, do breathing exercises, have a bath, or even talk with some friends. Surround yourself with positive people that don't drain you. Do something that soothes you. We all need to slow down and take some time for ourselves. Stress speeds up the aging process! Every moment you spend in a stressful state, you deplete valuable nutrients.

Nutrients are substances from food required by the human body to maintain vibrant health.[27] They are classified into two categories: macro-nutrients and micro-nutrients.[28] They are also considered substances essential for life-needed, bodily functions. Macro-nutrients are proteins, carbohydrates, fats, and water. Micro-nutrients are vitamins and minerals.

Carbohydrates are simple and complex sugars which deliver calories for energy. Simple carbohydrates are quickly digested. They consist of high calorie sugars like fructose (fruit), sucrose (table sugar), lactose (milk products), and glucose. Complex carbohydrates are slowly digested. They include starches like pasta, bread, grains, beans, potatoes, vegetables, and fiber. Starches are multiple combinations of simple sugars. They have more nutritional value than simple carbohydrates because they contain high vitamin and mineral content.

Fiber has no calories and the body doesn't readily digest it. We need approximately 25-30% of our daily calories from fiber. Fiber sweeps the digestive system free of unwanted substances that could promote cancer. It maintains bowel regularity, prevents disorders of the digestive tract, regulates blood sugar, and promotes a sense of fullness that may reduce overeating and unwanted weight gain.

Proteins are the main building materials for organs and muscles. Proteins that are complete contain all the essential amino acids in adequate amounts. They are lean meats, poultry, fish, tofu, low fat dairy, and eggs. Protein is crucial for growth, metabolism, and health. It is also the main structural element for skin, hair, nails, muscles, cell membranes, and connective tissues.

Collagen is skin protein which provides a barrier to foreign substances. Muscles are approximately 65% of the body's protein and they give the body strength and shape. We need 20 different proteins, nine of which are essential, meaning they cannot be made by our body and, therefore, must be obtained through food. There are eleven non-essential proteins and the body makes enough of them under normal circumstances.

Fat is the most concentrated form of food energy and contains approximately twice as many calories as carbohydrates and protein. We need approximately 20-30% of good fat in our daily calories. Fats include oils, butter, margarine, and nuts. They are needed to build cell membranes, make hormones (testosterone, estrogen, progesterone), insulation, and vital shock absorbers. A bit of advice...limit your saturated fat (animal fats-solid) intake.

Saturated fats are common in meat and dairy products. They are firm at room temperature. Mono- and poly-unsaturated fats (plant fats) are liquid at room temperature. These are good fats. Hydrogenated fats (trans fats) are solid at room temperature and you want to stay away from these! Sticks and tubs of margarine or butter, baked goods, and processed foods are examples of hydrogenated fats. Excess proteins, carbohydrates, and fats are converted and stored as fat! Micro-nutrients contain no calories (energy) and work with macro-nutrients for all processes. These are vitamins and minerals. The body requires approximately 13 essential vitamins and 22 essential trace mineral elements daily. These are the components that make enzymes work!! Don't forget to consult with a doctor or a physician before changing your diet or lifestyle.

Chapter 7
Cravings-What You Eat Affects How You Feel!!

If you haven't figured it out by now, there are certain foods that you eat which make you feel oh so good inside!! You get this calm feeling, or this burst of energy, as soon as it touches your tongue. Why does this happen? Well, here is the reason. There are a few chemicals and hormones in the body that can be directly linked to the food we eat.[29] They regulate body and brain processes, from your mood and what you want to eat to whether or not you experience headaches or develop a disease. Here are a few examples of these chemicals and their effects on our body.

Serotonin is called the mood regulator. High levels boost your mood, curb your food cravings, increase your pain tolerance, and help you sleep like a baby. On the other hand, low levels may cause insomnia, depression, food cravings, increased sensitivity to pain, and aggressive behavior. No other chemical is as strongly linked to your diet as serotonin. Eating a meal high in protein lowers serotonin levels, while eating a carbohydrate-rich snack has the opposite effects. When serotonin levels are high, this may cause an increased feeling of calmness or drowsiness, improves sleep patterns, increases pain tolerance, and reduces cravings for carbohydrate-rich foods. People who crave carbo-hydrates may suffer from an imbalance in serotonin. Carbo-hydrate-rich snacks make people feel better by curbing their craving and energizing them. People become conditioned to eat these foods when they feel tired, depressed or anx-ious. You must be able to choose the right types of carbo-hydrates to control this imbalance. If you completely elimi-nate carbohydrates from your diet, it could lead to an all out powerless binge. You don't want that! Complex, minimally processed carbohydrates are part of the solution. Try to stay away from simple carbohydrates such as sugar.

Dopamine and norepinephrine are the mood and en-ergy elevators. When these chemical's levels drop, you are likely to feel depressed, irritable, and moody. The amino acid that these chemicals are made from, are found in pro-tein-rich foods.

Acetylcholine is also known as the memory man-ager. Choline rich foods include wheat germ, soybeans, cauliflower, lentils, milk, potatoes, sesame seeds, barley, tomatoes, and egg yolks. Many of these foods contain not only choline but other forms of the nutrient including leci-thin. The choline is then converted to acetylcholine which is important in memory and general mental functioning. A deficit of acetylcholine is common with aging, memory loss, and reduces thinking, and possibly signs of Alzheimer's.

Everyone knows what endorphins are, right? The natural high we get from intense exercise, also called "run-ner's high," which causes endorphins to be released into the body. Some of us might not have experienced it, but we have heard about it. It is a feeling of joy and peacefulness that many athletes experience during and following exercise. Other pleasurable experiences raise the levels of endorphins such as laughter, soothing music, and meditation. The endorphins are your body's natural morphine-like chemicals that help boost your tolerance to pain, calm during stress, and produce feelings of euphoria and satisfaction. Endorphins don't encourage you to eat more and have no effect on our eating habits. They just make eating tasty, sweet, or creamy foods fun!! As I said earlier, sugar and fats just taste great!! Well endorphins are the reason for that. They make you "HAPPY"! When your levels of endorphins rise, it makes you want to eat more. Like that box of chocolate that you can't put down. Your desire for these creamy sweets increase. This is also related to the hormones of pregnancy and PMS which have you craving two weeks before your menstrual cycle.

Neuropeptide (NPY) along with blood-sugar levels, serotonin, and a couple of other chemicals, also determines your desire for carbohydrate-rich foods. Your levels of NPY raise up after waking from sleep. Because your body has been fasting overnight, this elevated level of NPY convinces you to eat waffles, pancakes, toast, jelly, doughnuts, and other carbohydrate-rich foods. Stress also triggers the release of NPY causing you to crave sweets. As you see, stress is one of the major forces that controls a lot of chemical reactions in the body. We talked about stress in the previous chapter and it was said that your thoughts are the number one acid producers in the body. We need to learn to control our thoughts so not to continue to damage our insides. As a professional athlete, I learned early in my career that competing at such a high level is approximately 85% mental. I had to learn to control my thoughts and think positive so that I would not be my worst enemy. You were already halfway defeated getting in the ring with a negative mindset.

Galanin is the chemical that has you craving fatty foods. When galanin levels rise, you desire foods such as salad dressing, chocolate, meat, ice cream, or potato chips. The breakdown of body fats during dieting, or when several hours go by without eating, releases these fats into the bloodstream. They are then taken to the brain which triggers a release of galanin causing you to crave these fat-containing foods. Simple isn't it?? There are other factors that cause the increase of this chemical. The reproductive hormone estrogen, stress hormone cortisol, and elevated insulin levels also cause galanin levels to increase. There-fore, we crave in times of stress, as well as times of PMS for women. Ladies, I think we have the short end of the stick!! So, we must be aware of the things we eat. Not just to maintain a good healthy weight, but also to maintain a healthy mood and demeanor. The food we put into our mouth, has an effect, one way or another, on our well-being, mind, body and soul.

Blood sugar controls your appetite and mood. Most hormones raise blood sugar levels when they fall be-low normal concentrations. Insulin balances the effects of these hormones by lowering blood sugar levels when they rise too high. When we digest the food we eat, our bod-ies break down sugars and starches into their simple units of glucose and fructose. The release of insulin is triggered when these simple units enter the blood stream. This insulin, with the help of nutrients (vitamins and minerals), supplies energy to tissues and maintains blood sugar levels. However, all carbohydrates are not created equal. Of course, unprocessed, complex carbohydrates are slowly broken down which produces a slow and progressive elevation in blood sugar. Processed starches, such as white bread or rice and concentrated sugars, are quickly broken down and trigger a larger release of insulin. This causes a dramatic drop in blood sugar to subnormal levels. The more often and the longer blood insulin levels remain high, the more likely a person is to accumulate excess body fat and battle a weight problem.

Food cravings are magnified when we diet, are under stress, when we skip meals, or are premenstrual. There is a biological connection between changes in body chemicals and food cravings. Food cravings also are fueled by an addiction to pleasure. It feels great to eat sweet and creamy foods. It brings us pleasure and a high from the endorphins. Food cravings are the body's way of telling you there may be a deficiency. If you can't eat something low fat and relatively healthy, the cravings may become more frequent. Most cravings fade within five to fifteen minutes.[30] There are plenty of fruits and vegetables that are sweet. Try these healthier options before you make other choices. We have heard the phrase, "sweet tooth." In reality, we crave fat. Most times we want chocolate, ice cream, and cookies. All of these have the same thing in common, sweetened FAT!!! Sugar just makes the fat taste better. Fat alone is not tasty. Sugar has a tendency to mask the fat in foods. Fat makes the food desirable and sugar makes the fat invisible.[31] Another important factor is smell. Fat carries many of the best aromas in food. The more turned on you are by the smell of foods, the more likely you are to battle food cravings. We are drawn to the sizzling steak, roasted turkey, and smell of bread baking. Fat makes food mouthwatering like the marbling in meat which makes it tender. You must resist the temptations of your senses and minimize these indulgences.

Over the years, I have tried all "fad" diets. When I say ALL, I mean ALL! I realized that all of the "diets" worked for a short time but they didn't sustain. They were just that...a "diet"...not a lifestyle change that I could continue to maintain or a way of life. They all literally manipulated the body to lose weight, for a lack of a better word. They created cravings because all of them, I found, were lacking in some area, which eventually created bingeing. I decided to modify my existing eating habits so that I could continue to follow it without "falling off the wagon", so to speak. People need to understand what works for them, that they can continue in a healthy way!

Chapter 8
Enzymes-Digestion

The digestion of food is largely taken for granted by everyone. More than $1 billion is spent annually on drugs to relieve heartburn, excess acid, bloating, and other symptoms of indigestion. These products are designed to give temporary relief from or mask these symptoms. They don't improve people's ability to digest food on their own.[32] More simply, the secret is that each raw, uncooked fruit, vegetable, or meat contains enzymes that will digest the food in which they are contained. The problem is that these enzymes are destroyed during cooking, canning, and other methods of food processing. Temperatures above 118 degrees Fahrenheit destroy the enzymes found in our food. We also eat food today that is processed (man-made) and contains no enzymes. When food enzymes are destroyed, your body may have to assume the entire burden of digesting food. This may cause health problems. When organs have to produce extra enzymes, this may cause them to enlarge and swell, requiring more tissue to make more secretions. This is another problem in itself! (That is another book!). Other minor problems may include food allergies, gas, bloating, heartburn, constipation, or diarrhea.

Now as we spoke earlier about food combining, this is very important to digestion. If digestion is slowed or incomplete, nutritional deficiencies could occur. Toxins that are deposited into the bloodstream may cause rashes, hives, headaches, nausea, and other symptoms commonly branded as allergies. And, as stated before, these symptoms are treated with drugs instead of trying to eat better! Do you see how this cycle of illness and taking drugs to mask the symptoms could continue to harm the body? Eating better for health is a process that is distinctive to every person. Do not change your daily routine without consulting with your doctor or physician before hand.

Hormones are some of the most powerful chemicals in the body. Special glands produce them (like the adrenals which produce adrenaline and the pancreas which produces insulin). Hormones are either fat-like, called steroid hormones, or protein-like, such as insulin. Hormone imbalances may wreak havoc on your health. Hormones are made from components of your food, so diet may play a crucial role in regulating your hormone balance.

Enzymes use vitamins and minerals from food to convert hormones into usable chemicals, so the body works properly. If any of these components (vitamins or minerals) are lacking, you may develop a deficiency and/or disease (e.g., osteoporosis, arthritis, etc.). Enzymes are in living things. Most enzymes are proteins secreted by cells that induce chemical changes.

"Enzymes are the construction workers of the body. They use the vitamins and minerals as building materials to put up the latest architectural marvel--your body. At times there is an ample supply of building material (nutrients with vitamins and minerals) but not enough workers (enzymes) to complete the job. The building materials will remain unused until enough workers show up at the site!"[33] This is a very significant statement.

Life is not possible without enzymes. Enzymes turn the food we eat into fuel for every single cell, be it a muscle cell, a brain cell, or a blood cell. Enzymes within these cells turn the fuel into usable energy that makes our heart beat, our nerves fire, and all other bodily functions take place. Vitamins and minerals make our life-giving enzymes function at their peak. All enzymes require the presence of water, the proper temperature and correct pH range in order to work. Enzymes digest food in the process of hydrolysis (the addition of water) to reduce food particles into smaller basic components. This is necessary for absorption.

Energy is defined as the capacity to do work. Enzymes are energy. They are the reason biochemical and physiological reactions occur in all living things. Enzymes are very important. The effectiveness of enzymes depends on the environment in which the enzyme acts. As we eat and digest food, the body releases enzymes from different organs to assist in the breakdown of food molecules. The nutrients are carried to other places by the blood to be used by the body to maintain wellness. This is linked to the acid-alkaline balance. In order for enzymes to work efficiently, they have to be in the right environment (meaning acidic or alkaline). Let me give you an example. Saliva contains an enzyme called ptyalin.[34] Its job is to breakdown large starch (complex carbohydrates) molecules into smaller ones to continue down the throat. It is said that Ptyalin works best in an alkaline environment (pH 6.5 or above). If the environment is acidic, its function may be hindered and so on and so forth. We will also talk about this in depth in another chapter.

Enzymes play an important role in keeping us healthy. Digestion relies on these enzymes to work their magic and breakdown food, giving us energy to move every day. Vitamins and minerals are not made by our bodies and we must consume them, in food or supplements, to possibly prevent deficiencies. They are the building blocks for enzymes to work effectively! Digestion starts in the mouth and continues on into the stomach. It takes up to one hour for your body to produce enough stomach acid to secrete enzymes for digestion to take place. This is only the beginning of digestion. It still has to go through the intestines, where possibly the liver, kidneys, pancreas, and bowels all continue to work (with enzymes) on food particles to get all the possible nutrients from it. How food is cooked also determines how well the body will use it.

Free-oxidizing radicals, sometimes called free radicals or oxidants, are the bad guys. They are produced by anything burnt, like a cigarette, sunlight, exhaust fumes, radiation, fried fat, or burnt meat. This is the body equivalent of nuclear waste. They are harmful and may damage your body. Normal processes generate oxygen radicals and the body has a system of enzymes and antioxidants to combat them. When these defense mechanisms are overwhelmed, free radical damage takes place and degenerative disease may begin. This damage may, in the long run, lead to cancer, inflammation, aging, and arterial damage.

Antioxidants are like flame-proof gloves that can disarm potential damaging properties of free radicals. Antioxidants are enzymes that have specific missions to search and destroy free radicals. Similarly, there are antioxidants that neutralize free radicals and may, over time, prevent and even reverse the effects of some diseases, whose primary cause is excess oxidation. Our food sources of polyunsaturated, fatty acids easily bond to oxygen and form free radicals. But, antioxidants move in and neutralize them. Some antioxidants are known as essential nutrients like vitamin A, and beta carotene. Other antioxidants, like bioflavonoids, are not essential. A few examples of antioxidants that work in the body are Vitamins A, C, E, Zinc, Selenium, and CoQ10.

The balance between your intake of antioxidants and your exposure to free radicals may be the balance between good and bad health! Simple changes in your diet and supplementing antioxidants can tip the scales in your favor. In addition, these changes may reduce the production of free radicals that damage our bodies. Some foods that contain antioxidants are carrots, peaches, mangoes, papayas, cantaloupes, sweet potatoes, spinach, and parsley. Consult your doctor or physician before taking supplements.

Chapter 9
Protein--How much is enough? Too much?

We need protein. Protein is made up of 25 amino acids.[35] Proteins make approximately 75% of the solid parts of our body.[36] Enzymes and hormones are primarily proteins. Protein is instrumental in most of the functions of the body. It is suggested that the best quality proteins are eggs, meat, fish, beans, lentils, soybeans and quinoa. Animal protein contains undesirable fats; vegetable proteins contain additional beneficial complex carbohydrates and are less acid forming. However, its been said that the protein in meat is more usable than the protein in plants. If we get our protein from a variety of sources, we will get more of the 25 amino acids that we need. I recommend, when eating meat, make sure it's organic and the leanest part or cut. It makes a difference considering all the hormones and pesticides contained in food these days. I started buying organic products, as much as possible, to minimize the chemicals I ingested daily. I have noticed a difference over time in my daily routine, as well as, my athletic performance. The irony is that protein is not only essential but also potentially health-destroying in excess.

The consumption of excess dietary protein may congest your cells and forces the pH of your life-sustaining fluids down to disease producing levels. Excessive amounts of protein may cause toxicity. Meat eaters are likely to visit the doctor or be admitted to the hospital twice as often as a vegetarians.[37] Excess protein is said to be a contributor to osteoporosis, over-acidity, and many other common health problems. When our bodies neutralize the over-acidity, sodium and calcium are affected. Over-acidity may cause calcium depletion in the bones, which may cause an increased risk of osteoporosis. In women, estrogen assists in retaining calcium in bones. Menopause ceases the production of estrogen. Women may be at an even greater risk of osteoporosis if they are not getting enough calcium from their foods or taking supplements.

The kidneys become overworked when excess protein exists in the body. This may cause deteriorated kidney function. It may also lead to an increase in kidney stone formation, decreased calcium balance, and you may be at risk for bone loss. Protein is an energy producer. However, it takes more energy to digest it than to generate it. Therefore, it is a negative energy source. Protein takes longer to digest. The feeling of more energy from protein lasts longer.

Protein doesn't increase energy, it stimulates! Let me explain. "Nervous energy" – fidgety foot bouncers, finger tappers, and channel changers – manifests symptoms of excess protein consumption. Nervous energy is misunderstood as actual energy when, in reality, it may be overstimulation. Protein is second to prescription drugs as a major stimulant![38] Even coffee, tea, and sodas are weak sisters compared to protein. Caffeine drinks don't have anywhere near the stimulatory staying power of a steak! These drinks are stimulants for only an hour or so. Protein may keep you hyped for several hours. This is why some people are up all night after eating a major protein meal for dinner.

The body takes a long time to digest protein and it is revved up for hours. I have experienced this a few times after eating a high protein meal before I "tried" to go to sleep. It was not happening! As the body sleeps, rebuilding takes place but it can't do it properly if it is over-stimulated. As more acid-producing protein is consumed, sodium may be taken from the alkaline reserves to neutralize this acid. When the body steals alkaline reserves and they are drained, it may eventually take from other sources. We need approximately 30-35 grams of protein daily, unless you are performing excessive exercise or recovering from surgery. The myth that extra protein is needed to make stronger and bigger muscles, is just that, a myth!

Muscle is only approximately 22% protein, so an increased intake of 2-3 grams a day will bring about the greatest possible muscle gain. Any more than this may be transformed into fat for storage and become taxing on the body from toxicity! Protein contains nitrogen. Nitrogen isn't the bad guy. We need nitrogen. We can eliminate nitrogen as urea (neutralized salt formed by the liver) through our urine, however, too much protein may cause accumulation and signal the reserves to kick into action. As it gets worse and reserves are drained, ammonia becomes the product eliminated through the urine.

Ammonia is the waste product of nitrogen. The odor

of ammonia in urine is a possible signal that the body is responding to an emergency of too little sodium. People who suffer from gout (painful inflammation of joints due to excess uric acid in the blood from excess protein) may be familiar with this. Pain or burning when you urinate may be an indication that the reserves of neutralizing minerals are exhausted and the body has adapted the way it functions for survival, not comfort! A possible way to improve this condition is to eat foods that will replenish the supply of neutralizing minerals--the alkaline reserves, meaning fruits and vegetables.

Chapter 10
Acid-Alkaline Balance

Nutrition is a very important part of our life. Ninety percent of our wellness starts from within. What you put in (food, nutrition, fuel) is what you get out (energy, wellness, illness, appearance). The energy produced from a small amount of the right food powers all processes. In order for the body's cells to function properly, they need to receive life-giving nutrients and oxygen from the bloodstream and to release waste. For these processes to optimally take place, the body must be in a slightly alkaline state. I'm going to take you back to a refresher course in high school chemistry! I know many of us have been out of school for years, but bear with me. Alkaline and acidic states are the pH of the body. The term pH stands for "potential of Hydrogen." pH is measured on a scale of 0-14, with 7 being neutral, lower than 7 is acidic, and higher than 7 is alkaline.

Proper acid-alkaline balance is one of the most essential elements of optimal health, as I have found out. Let me repeat that statement! Proper acid-alkaline balance is one of the most essential elements of optimal health! If you haven't heard anything at all in this book, please listen to this chapter very carefully. It will give you some very good information that I found very useful to me in my journey. Small changes in pH readings represent major changes in body functions. Potassium (one of the body's electrolytes) is an alkalizing element. It plays one of the most important roles in maintaining the acid-alkaline balance in the body. Another important electrolyte is chloride which, together with sodium (organic salt from the food we eat, not table salt), acts to stabilize the pH of the blood. Disproportionate loss of chloride can lead to the body's environment becoming more acidic, therefore possibly leading to health problems.

The body is alkaline by design and acid producing by function. The body's metabolic processes, like breathing, movement and the beating of your heart, produce lots of acid. In order for them to work, they need to be in an alkaline environment. The body is able to deal with and eliminate the acid that is produced by metabolic processes. However, it is overwhelmed from the acid produced by some of the food we eat. Because of its ingenious construction and function, the body works overtime to correct this process of over-acidity. So how does the body maintain its balance? The food we eat is the deciding factor whether our body will be acidic or alkaline. Research says, the average American diet normally consists of more acidic foods. Of the four food groups – meats, dairy, fruits and vegetables, and grains – meats, dairy, and grains are acid producing foods. Alkaline foods consist of fruits, vegetables, and spices. It is recomended that you incorporate plenty of fruits and vegetables in every meal for the body to maintain a healthy balance and optimal internal processes.

The majority of foods at every meal should be alkalizing. If the body is more acidic, the body neutralizes the acid with fluid. This is why it is necessary to consume enough fluid. The first body part to help neutralize the acid is the kidneys. Next is the lungs and then skin to excrete the excess acid. Excess acid is eliminated through the kidneys and bowels but they need to be neutralized. If it isn't neutralized, it could possibly burn tissues as it exited. Sometimes the muscles are affected. For example, fluid around and in the bone is taken if the problem calls for even more fluid to neutralize the acid. This may cause osteoarthritis. Possible ways to improve the condition is to eat foods that will replenish the supply of neutralizing minerals (alkaline reserve).

Your alkaline reserve is comprised of minerals that offset the effects of dietary acid. These minerals are calcium, sodium, potassium and magnesium. They are found, in abundance, in fruits and vegetables. You must replenish these alkaline reserves constantly or they will vanish quickly, as the body needs to compensate most of the time. There are alternative sources of these minerals, such as your bones, which contain calcium. Calcium's principle job is to keep your bones solid!! So, you see, there is a process to fixing internal problems that the body uses before symptoms develop from another problem due to the initial tilt the of acid-alkaline balance (e.g., osteoarthritis).

The body is smart and, without thought from you, it saves you pain and discomfort everyday. To what extent, though, are we willing to compromise our insides for our body to keep making up for our mistakes? Nutrients play an important role in good health. Your body may not last as long without the proper nutrients. Your body is able to fully absorb and make use of nutrients only within specific pH levels. A healthy range is 7.36-7.45.[39] If not, a number of problems may result and nutritional deficiencies follow. A tip about carbonated soft drinks...carbonated soft drinks are among the most acidifying substances found in the super-market. Research shows that in order to neutralize one glass of soda, the average person needs to drink thirty two glasses of water![40] WOW! How many sodas have you had in the last day or two? I know I have cut down tremendously.

Let's talk briefly about antacids. Antacids are used to relieve heartburn – one of the more common side effects of a highly acidifying diet. Heartburn tends to happen when acid from your stomach backs up into your esophagus (throat). People mistake heartburn as too much acid. In reality, it's too little acid and the stomach cannot produce good, quality mucus to protect itself. Although antacids are used to neutralize heartburn, they may make it worse. This may lead to undigested food particles which ferment inside the stomach. Again, this can cause inflammation, irritation, bloating, digestive pain, and other digestive problems. The body is very complicated and we need to take these little tips into consideration. Many of them are linked to each other in some way or another.

Everything we talk about when it comes to food, health, and nutrition always refers back to the subject of pH. This is the major premise to how the body operates at optimum levels. Everything from enzymes, digestion, use of water, energy, food, etc. are all predicated on the acid-alkaline balance inside our body for these processes to work properly. Foods can also be considered expansive or contractive. Expansive foods are foods that temporarily stimulate like coffee, sugar, alcohol, drugs, and chocolate. Contractive foods have a restricting effect. Examples are proteins, dairy products, and salt. The body must devote a lot of attention to processing both these types of foods. Neutral foods are fruits, vegetables, grains, seeds, beans, and nuts. Expansive and contractive foods are stressful to the body. Understand this…if you consume a lot of one (e.g., alcohol), you will probably crave the other (e.g., salt). The body is a balance seeking mechanism. For example, wine and cheese go together just like beer and pretzels. The body has its ways of telling you that something is wrong! We just need to pay attention.

Chapter 11
Finale

The secret to being healthy is to know which foods do what and balance the two kinds, so your body can function at its best. You do not need to be a vegetarian to be healthy. It's a matter of choice. When you eat more fruits and vegetables than acid producing foods, like meats, breads, and pastas, your body can maintain the necessary reserves, therefore allowing vitamins and minerals to perform their functions. As a result, good health is sure to follow. When you realize that the food you put in your mouth has an effect on your cells (the foundation of your physical being), it presents a whole different view of eating.

Eating serves an infinitely, more important function than being merely an exercise in fellowship (socially) or satisfaction of appetite. One way to identify nutritional needs for enzymes is to conduct a urinalysis exam. The exam detects what is being eliminated through the kidneys and bladder. It tells us what our bodies are throwing away due to having too much and what it is holding on to because of a deficiency. There are different tests to identify vitamin and mineral analysis.[41] They tell us what we get enough of and what we need more of. Some include hair analysis, blood tests, urine tests, sweat and taste, and food intolerance tests. Another way that is recommended to get on the right track is to do a cleansing or a detoxification program. I can't stress this point enough...make sure you receive consultation from a professional (nutritionist, dietician, or doctor) before you begin a detoxification, cleansing, or any of the analysis tests.

Don't expect exercise to take off pounds if too much of the wrong kind of food is going into your mouth. I hear it all the time. "If I exercise, I can eat anything right?" WRONG! It doesn't work that way. You might look good on the outside. But what do you look like on the inside? Health and wellness start from within. I tell this to everyone interested in getting back into "shape." You have to do it right because fitness and nutrition go hand in hand, with nutrition being the most important, as I have learned.

Let's all take time to make our health a priority so we can all live a better life. Do it for yourself! This will improve your confidence and strengthen you to do whatever you want to do in life. It doesn't hurt to try. But it does hurt to be sick and full of disease when we are supposed to live life to the fullest. For you to be healthy, you must provide your body with enough natural nutrients to keep your cells healthy. It's your health--it's your choice.

In the next few pages, I will highlight a few tips that are important to me and that I have incorporated over the years. They will help you make better choices. I hope these are useful to you and help you get on the right track, slowly, living a more fulfilled and healthy life as it has for me.

Thank you to all who supported me in buying this

book and had the confidence in me to give you some of my knowledge and experience to help you. If this was good useful information, please refer it to a friend or family member so you can help them get on track, too! I encourage you to get out and exercise a little each day for the purpose of staying in good shape (strength and posture). It helps your heart muscle to work more efficiently. It can't hurt, it only helps. Please consult your doctor or physician before starting a new program relating to health, fitness, and wellness.

Thanks, Isra Girgrah Wynn.

Appendix A
50 Nutritional Tips for Your Everyday Life

1.   Make healthy choices. When you sit down at home or at a restaurant, think about the choices you are about to make. Instead of that fried chicken, eat baked chicken. Instead of french fries, try a garden salad. It can make a huge difference.

2.   Eat small frequent meals. Try eating 6-7 smaller meals each day instead of the traditional 3 big meals. This will speed up your metabolism and allow you to maintain a healthier weight.

3.   Eat regular meals. Don't veer off the plan of eating at specific times because it causes bingeing and/or overeating. Don't eat unless you are hungry.

4.   Don't wait too long before eating. Once you have waited too long between meals your body's blood sugar levels go haywire. Try not to wait longer than 4 hours between meals. You will also cut down on bingeing.

5.   Practice portion control. When you eat, make sure you are not piling the food onto your plate. The eyes are always bigger than the stomach. Limit yourself to smaller portions. This will allow your body to digest better and not stretch your stomach out.

6.   Don't confuse fat-free with calorie-free. Fat-free foods still have a lot of sugar and that, in itself, has a lot of calories attached to it. These are bad foods in disguise.

7.   Don't deprive yourself. If you have a craving, satisfy it. Try not to eat the whole cake or the whole carton of candy!! Just have enough to satisfy that craving and then continue with your healthy eating.

8.   Stop eating when you're satisfied, not full. You know those times when you can't push away from the table! Once you are satisfied, stop eating. You can always come back to it later. It won't go anywhere! It's not the last meal that you will ever eat.

9.   Give your body a chance to feel full. Eat slowly. Your body takes approximately 20 minutes to realize that it is full! Eat slow so you can give it time to figure it out. Say a whole sentence between bites to slow you down.

10.   Eat anti-stress foods. If you are feeling stressed, eat your fruit with some nuts or brown rice with fish. Nuts, seeds, beans, and lentils already contain both protein and carbohydrates and are, therefore, good anti-stress foods.

11.   Fast-releasing sugars create a state of stress on the body, stimulating the release of cortisol (makes fatty acids). Avoid eating white bread, sweets, and breakfast cereals or other foods with added sugar.

12.   How much protein is enough? Ten to fifteen percent of your daily calories are suggested because you get protein from other foods which add up during the day. Too much is toxic.

13.   Margarine is one of the worst processed food you can put in your body. The oils have been mutilated and hydrogenated; it's a phony food.

14.   Cravings are associated with acid-alkaline imbalances. When you start eating healthier and have more balanced meals, you will curb your cravings. This is due to the acid-alkaline fluid being balanced inside your body.

15.   Cooking strengthens bonds of certain food and destroys enzymes. This makes it harder to break down and digest. Your system doesn't get the benefit from these cooked foods as it would raw foods.

16.   There are two specific times it is suggested you should not eat...when you are not hungry and when you have a fever above 100 degrees. During the latter, the body is cleaning. Just drink water (fluid).

17.   A breakfast of fruit is an ideal way to start your day. It is light, easily digested and provides energy to start your day right.

18.   A protein meal should be the last meal of the day. It

takes longer to digest and it is a negative energy food. It takes a lot of energy to process protein.

19.   The brain is one of the largest consumers of DHA. DHA is an essential fatty acid (omega 3). You can get this from certain fish oils. It is said that the adult brain consists of more than 20 grams of DHA!

20.   Hydrochloric acid (produced in stomach) declines in old age. The consequence is indigestion, particularly after high-protein meals and the likelihood of food allergies might occur.

21.   Raw vegetables have a thin coating called cellulose which protects them. The body doesn't digest this. If we don't remove this thin layer while chewing, we will develop gas. The enzyme found in vegetables, cellulase, helps with digestion and has to be released beyond that thin layer. Chew your vegetables well.

22.   The addition of organic calcium prevents muscle cramps. Try two oranges a day to avoid and prevent muscle cramps.

23.   Fruits and vegetables have all the nutrients your cells need to keep them producing energy. The fresher, the better.

24.   The sweeter the vegetable, no matter what region they are grown in, the more it contains all the nutrients we were meant to have. Bitter vegetables lack needed nutri-

ents. It is not recommended to drink bitter vegetable juice either.

25.   Soy protein is hard to digest because it contains the highest concentration if enzyme inhibitors which need certain conditions to activate the enzymes. Enzyme inhibitors are in most seeds and grains.

26.   It is highly not recommended to exercise after a big meal (especially acid forming foods-protein). Large protein meals generate acid and aerobic exercise generates even more acid!! Acid on top of acid can raise the acid in your body to disastrous levels!!

27.   Walking, when done right, may help with symptoms of headache sufferers. Swing the arms opposite the legs and walk at a good pace. The arm movement is key. It's the contralateral movement of the opposite arm and leg that may relieve the headache.

28.   It is not recommended to take B vitamins late at night if you have difficulty sleeping.

29.   It has been said that women with poor diets are particularly at risk for morning sickness when pregnant.

30.   It is suggested that you increase your Vitamin C intake to 3 grams every four hours to fight infection (colds).

31.   Difficulty building muscle is rarely due to a lack of

protein. It is often a result of not taking enough muscle building vitamins and minerals, such as zinc and vitamin B6, which helps digest and use dietary protein.

32.   Aerobic exercise adds years to your lifespan where anaerobic exercise promotes better cardiovascular (heart) health. Try to incorporate both into your daily plan with consultation from your doctor.

33.   Graze don't gorge! The excess food we eat is converted into fat and stored.

34.   Cooking changes the molecules in food and destroys many valuable nutrients and the enzymes that break food down into components to be used by the body.

35.   Protein and sugar together (for example, ice cream) is said to be one of the worst combinations. It causes havoc inside the body.

36.   Liquids, including water, dilute digestive fluids; they should not be consumed during meals. Before and after is recommended.

37.   Supplements serve a useful purpose when taken occasionally. They don't make you healthy. You should try to get most of your vitamins and minerals from a variety of healthy foods.

38.   Balance is the key to a healthy body, attitude, and

personality.

39.   There is a lot of calcium in milk, but it is not usable!! Pasteurization changes the structure of milk. It is suggested that the best calcium you can get is from fruits and vegetables.

40.   We were designed to eat foods grown in nature, not foods adulterated or "improved" by man. It has been said that many symptoms of major illnesses may be indirect effects of a deficiency of dietary organic sodium (from fruits and vegetables, not table salt).

41.   More than half the nutrients in the food you eat are destroyed before they reach your plate, depending on the food you choose, how you store it, and how you cook it.

42.   Eat as much raw food as possible, with the exception of meat, poultry, and fish. Steam food where you can, and fry as little as possible or avoid it all together. Buy organic foods and eat whole foods instead of refined and processed foods.

43.   Fizzy drinks containing phosphorus can inhibit calcium absorption as can drinks containing caffeine. One that contains both is bad news (for example, sodas).

44.   Exercising makes the blood more acidic, and deep breathing makes it more alkaline.

45.   It is recommended that you don't start your day with a stimulant (coffee, tea, cigarette), because the "stress" state inhibits digestion.

46.   Meats, eggs, cheese, refined grains, and wheat (which contain gluten) are all constipating foods. Eating plenty of fruits, vegetables, and whole grains, plus drinking water, is essential in combating this.

47.   Balancing blood sugar levels (with protein and/or fats in your meal) is the key to appetite and weight control. This will control blood sugar from rising and storing excess as fat.

48.   Good food should be low in fat, salt, and fast-releasing sugars; high in fiber, and alkaline forming. Non-animal protein (vegetable) is desirable. Choose foods low in calories.

49.   A craving for food when you have already eaten enough calories is often a craving for more nutrients, so foods providing "empty" calories should be strictly avoided.

50.   We live and die at the cellular level. When your cells are in trouble, you are too!!

Appendix B
Meal Plan Choices - Breakfast

Breakfast # 1
1 cup cooked oatmeal with water or low fat milk
Fruit
Tea (Herbal)

Breakfast # 2
Whole Grain muffin
Fruit
Tea (herbal)

Breakfast # 3
3 eggs (1 whole egg, 2 egg whites)
1 ounce low Fat Cheese
2 Slices of whole wheat toast
Fruit
Juice

Breakfast # 4
2 Whole Wheat waffles
Fruit
Low fat Milk

Breakfast # 5
2 Pancakes (whole wheat)
Fruit
Tea (Herbal) or Juice

Breakfast # 6
1 cup low fat Granola
Fruit
Tea (Herbal) or Juice

Breakfast # 7
1 cup low Fat Yogurt
Fruit
Tea (Herbal) or Juice

Breakfast # 8
3/4 cup whole Grain Cereal
Low Fat Milk

Breakfast # 9
3/4 cup low Fat Cottage Cheese
Fruit
Tea (Herbal)

Breakfast # 10
3 Egg Omelette (1 whole egg, 2 egg whites)
Vegetables
Slice of Whole Wheat Toast
Tea (Herbal) or Low Fat Milk

Appendix C
Meal Plan Choices - Lunch

Lunch # 1
Whole Wheat Pita Pocket
2 ounces low Fat Cheese
Vegetables
Water (Still or Sparkling) with lemon or lime

Lunch # 2
1 cup tuna Salad (low fat dressing)
Vegetables
Water (Still or Sparkling) with Lemon or lime

Lunch # 3
1 cup grilled Chicken Salad (low fat dressing)
Variety of Vegetables
Water (Still or Sparkling) with Lemon or lime

Lunch # 4
1 cup soup (broth based-low sodium and fat)
Water or Low Fat Milk

Lunch # 5
Vegetable Pizza (6 inches in diameter)
Water or Low Fat Milk

Lunch # 6
Tomato and Low Fat Cheese

2 Slices of Whole Wheat Toast
Water or Low Fat Milk

Lunch # 7
Salad (Variety of Vegetables)
Low Fat Dressing (sparingly)
Shrimp (8-10 pieces, medium)
Water or Low Fat Milk

Lunch # 8
Bean Salad
Water or Tea (Herbal)

Lunch # 9
2 Slices of Whole Wheat Toast
Sliced Roasted Turkey (3-4 slices)
Tea (Herbal) or Low Fat Milk

Lunch # 10
Turkey Patty (3 ounces)
Salad
Tea (Herbal) or Low Fat Milk

Appendix D
Meal Plan Choices - Dinner

Dinner # 1
Grilled Salmon (3-5 ounces)
Vegetables (Grilled or Steamed)
Water or Tea (Herbal)

Dinner # 2
3/4 cup Whole Wheat Rice
Vegetables (Grilled or Steamed)
1/2 cup potatoes
Water or Tea (Herbal)

Dinner # 3
Grilled or Roast Chicken Breast (3 ounces)
Vegetables (Grilled or Steamed)
Tea (Herbal) or Water

Dinner # 4
3/4 cup Whole Wheat Pasta
Vegetables (Grilled or Steamed)
Low Fat Cream Sauce

Dinner # 5
Steak (4 ounces)
Vegetables (Grilled or Steamed)
Water or Tea (Herbal)

Dinner # 6
Grilled or Broiled Fish (Halibut, Tilapia) (3-5 ounces)
Vegetables (Grilled or Steamed)
Water or Tea (Herbal)

Dinner # 7
Vegetable Pizza (6 inches diameter)
Salad
Water or Tea (Herbal)

Dinner # 8
Chicken Stir Fry (3 ounces)
Vegetables (Variety)
Tea (Herbal)

Dinner # 9
Roasted Potatoes (3/4 cup)
Variety of Vegetables Grilled or Steamed
Tea (Herbal) or Water (Still or Sparkling)

Dinner # 10
Burrito (Corn)
Chicken or Steak (Grilled) (3 ounces)
Vegetables
Tea (Herbal) or Water (Still or Sparkling)

Appendix E
Meal Plan Choices - Snacks

Snack # 1
Fruit
Nuts

Snack # 2
Popcorn
Low Fat Butter

Snack # 3
Tortilla Chips
Salsa or Bean Dip or Low fat Cheese dip

Snack # 4
Whole Wheat Pretzel
Mustard

Snack # 5
Apples
Peanut Butter

Snack # 6
Yogurt
Fruit

Snack # 7
Strawberries
Low Fat Chocolate Sauce (preferably Dark chocolate)

Snack # 8
Low Fat Cheese
Whole Wheat Crackers

Snack # 9
Vegetables
Dip (Low Fat Ranch)

Snack # 10
Slice of Whole Wheat Toast
Low Fat Cream Cheese

Snack # 11
Fruit Smoothy

Snack # 12
Mixed nuts
Dried Fruit

Snack # 13
Fig Bars

Snack # 14
Sorbet
Fruit

Snack # 15
Shrimp
Cocktail sauce

Note: Any meal can be seasoned with any herb or seasoning except salt!! Salt should be limited.

Your average daily caloric intake is as follows: most women and older adults, approximately 1600-1800; teen girls, active women, and most men, approximately 2200-2600; teen boys, and active men approximately 2600-3000. These daily averages depend on your level of activity.

Please consult with your doctor or a physician before you change your lifestyle with respect to health and fitness.

About the Author

Isra Girgrah Wynn grew up in Canada for most of her life. She attended Queen's University in Ontario, Canada and studied biology as her major, with a minor in health. As the years passed, she gravitated more towards health. Upon moving to Washington DC, she pursued a professional boxing career and competed for 10 years. She met her husband, Marty Wynn, along the way. They have been happily married for 10 years and have 4 beautiful children.

Isra has always been interested in her own health and wellness, and the health and wellness of others. She is a personal fitness and boxing trainer and a nutrition consultant. She advises clients interested in making life changes. She continues to educate herself and increase her knowledge by taking health and fitness courses. Isra has taken courses in Holistic Nutrition and Herbology over the last 5 years. As a full-time mother and wife, she is concerned about the wellness of her family. As a driven champion, Isra's passion motivates her to continue the pursuit of optimum health and nutrition. Isra hopes that her journey will help others achieve a positive state of wellness and make their health a priority.

Isra is certain that, with a few health and nutrition

tips, people can start making small changes to feel better, which will make a big difference in the long run. This book outlines these tips and small bits of information, making its readers more aware of how our brilliant bodies function and how to make steps to live a pain- and illness-free life.

Glossary of Terms

acetylcholine - a compound that occurs throughout the nervous system, in which it functions as a neurotransmitter

acid - a compound usually having a sour taste and capable of neutralizing alkalis and reddening blue litmus paper

adrenaline (also known as epinephrine) - a hormone secreted by the adrenal medulla upon stimulation by the central nervous system in response to stress, as anger or fear, and acting to increase heart rate, blood pressure, cardiac output, and carbohydrate metabolism

Alzheimer's - a disease marked by progressive loss of mental capacity

arthritis - inflammation of a joint, usually accompanied by pain, swelling, and stiffness, and resulting from infection, trauma, degenerative changes, metabolic disturbances, or other causes. It occurs in various forms, such as bacterial arthritis, osteoarthritis, or rheumatoid arthritis

bacteria - a very large group of microorganisms comprising one of the three domains of living organisms

calories - a unit equal to the kilocalorie, used to express the heat output of an organism and the fuel or energy value of food

chemicals - narcotic or mind-altering drugs or substances

choline - a strongly basic compound occurring widely in living tissues and important in the synthesis and transport of lipids (fats)

collagen - the fibrous protein constituent of bone, cartilage, tendon, and other connective tissue

deficient - lacking an essential quality or element; insufficient, inadequate in amount

degenerative disease - a disease characterized by progressive degenerative changes in tissue

dehydration - an abnormal loss of water from the body, especially from illness or physical exertion

detoxification - the metabolic process by which toxins are changed into less toxic or more readily excretable substances

diabetes - any of several metabolic disorders marked by excessive discharge of urine and persistent thirst, especially one of the two types of diabetes mellitus

diet - the usual food and drink of a person

digestion - the process by which food is converted into substances that can be absorbed and assimilated by the body disease - a pathological condition of a part, organ, or system of an organism resulting from various causes, such as infection, genetic defect, or environmental stress, and characterized by an identifiable group of signs or symptoms

diuretic - a substance that increases the rate of urine production

dopamine - a neurotransmitter formed in the brain, essential to the normal functioning of the central nervous system

drug - a substance used in the diagnosis, treatment, or prevention of a disease or as a component of a medication

endorphins - any of a group of peptide hormones that bind to opiate receptors and are found mainly in the brain

energy - the capacity for doing work

enzymes - any of numerous complex proteins that are produced by living cells and catalyze specific biochemical reactions at body temperatures

essential - a substance that is required for normal functioning but cannot be synthesized by the body and therefore must be included in the diet

fecal matter (feces) - waste product from the digestive tract

ferment - to cause agitation or excitement

fitness - good health or physical condition; especially as the result of exercise and proper nutrition

galanin - a neurotransmitter that plays a role in regulating various physiological functions and is thought to be associated with the urge to eat fatty foods

glucose - a simple sugar; the living cell uses it as a source of energy

health - a condition of optimal well-being; soundness, especially of body or mind; freedom from disease or abnormality

homeostasis - the ability or tendency of an organism or a cell to maintain internal equilibrium by adjusting its physiological processes

hormones - a chemical messenger that carries a signal from one cell to another

illness - poor health resulting from disease of body or mind; sickness

insulin - a hormone secreted by the pancreas that regulates the levels of sugar in the blood

metabolism - the chemical processes occurring within a living cell or organism that are necessary for the maintenance of life neuropeptide (NPY) - any group of compounds that act as neurotransmitters and are short chain polypeptides

neurotransmitters - a chemical substance that is released at the end of a nerve fiber by the arrival of a nerve impulse

neutralize - to put out of action or make incapable of action

non-essential - a substance required for normal functioning but not needed in the diet because the body can synthesize it

norepinephrine - a hormone that is released by the adrenal medulla and by the sympathetic nerves and functions as a neurotransmitter

nutrient - a source of nourishment, especially a nourishing ingredient in a food

nutrition - the process of nourishing or being nourished, especially the process by which a living organism assimilates food and uses it for growth and for replacement of tissues

optimum - the point at which the condition, degree, or amount of something is the most favorable

osteoporosis - a disorder in which the bones become increasingly porous, brittle, and subject to fracture, owing to loss of calcium and other mineral components

oxidation - the combination of a substance with oxygen

pancreas - a gland, situated near the stomach, that secretes a digestive fluid into the intestine through one or more ducts and also secretes the hormone insulin

putrefaction - the anaerobic decomposition of organic matter by bacteria and fungi that results in obnoxiously odorous products; rotting

rancid - a decomposition process in food

secretion - the act or process of separating, elaborating, and releasing a substance that fulfills some function within the organism or undergoes excretion

serotonin - a neurotransmitter, derived from tryptophan, that is involved in sleep, depression, memory, and other neurological processes

stimulant - an agent, especially a chemical agent such as caffeine, that temporarily arouses or accelerates physiological or organic activity

symptom - a sign or an indication of disorder or disease, especially when experienced by an individual as a change from normal function, sensation, or appearance

toxin - a poisonous substance, especially protein, that is produced by living cells or organisms and is capable of causing disease when introduced into the body tissues but is often also capable of inducing neutralizing antibodies or antitoxins

wealth - an abundance or profusion of anything; plentiful
amount

Notes

1. Morter, M.T. (2000). Fells Official Know-It-All-Guide: Health & Wellness. Hollywood, FL: Frederick Fell Publishers, Inc.

2. Holford, P. (2004). The New Optimum Nutrition Bible. Berkeley, CA: Crossing Press

3. Holford, P. (2004). The New Optimum Nutrition Bible. Berkeley, CA: Crossing Press

4. Holford, P. (2004). The New Optimum Nutrition Bible. Berkeley, CA: Crossing Press

5. Holford, P. (2004). The New Optimum Nutrition Bible. Berkeley, CA: Crossing Press

6. Institute of Natural Medicine. Holistic Nutrition. Chevy Chase, MD.

7. Institute of Natural Medicine. Holistic Nutrition. Chevy Chase, MD.

8. Institute of Natural Medicine. Holistic Nutrition. Chevy Chase, MD.

9. Institute of Natural Medicine. Holistic Nutrition. Chevy Chase, MD.

10. Somer, E. (1999). Food & Mood. New York, NY: Henry Holt and Company, LLC.

11. Batmanghelidj, F. (1995). Your Body's Many Cries For Water. Vienna, VA: Global Health Solutions, Inc.

12. Walker, R. (2007). The Human Body Book (S. Parker, Ed.). New York, NY: Dorling Kindersley Publishing

13. Walker, R. (2007). The Human Body Book (S. Parker, Ed.). New York, NY: Dorling Kindersley Publishing

14. Holford, P. (2004). The New Optimum Nutrition Bible. Berkeley, CA: Crossing Press

15. Holford, P. (2004). The New Optimum Nutrition Bible. Berkeley, CA: Crossing Press

16. Holford, P. (2004). The New Optimum Nutrition Bible. Berkeley, CA: Crossing Press

17. Batmanghelidj, F. (1995). Your Body's Many Cries For Water. Vienna, VA: Global Health Solutions, Inc.

18. Batmanghelidj, F. (1995). Your Body's Many Cries For Water. Vienna, VA: Global Health Solutions, Inc.

19. Batmanghelidj, F. (1995). Your Body's Many Cries For Water. Vienna, VA: Global Health Solutions, Inc.

20. Loomis, H.F. (2005). Enzymes, The Key to Health, Volume 1: The Fundamentals. Madison, WI: Grote Publishing

21. Loomis, H.F. (2005). Enzymes, The Key to Health, Volume 1: The Fundamentals. Madison, WI: Grote Publishing

22. Brown, S.E., & Trivieri, L. (2006). The Acid-Alkaline Food Guide: A Quick Reference to Foods & Their Effect on pH Levels. Garden City Park, NY: Square One Publishers

23. Holford, P. (2004). The New Optimum Nutrition Bible. Berkeley, CA: Crossing Press

24. Holford, P. (2004). The New Optimum Nutrition Bible. Berkeley, CA: Crossing Press

25. Morter, M.T. (2000). Fells Official Know-It-All-Guide: Health & Wellness. Hollywood, FL: Frederick Fell Publishers, Inc.

26. Holford, P. (2004). The New Optimum Nutrition Bible. Berkeley, CA: Crossing Press

27. Institute of Natural Medicine. Holistic Nutrition. Chevy Chase, MD.

28. Institute of Natural Medicine. Holistic Nutrition. Chevy Chase, MD.

29. Somer, E. (1999). Food & Mood. New York, NY: Henry Holt and Company, LLC.

30. Somer, E. (1999). Food & Mood. New York, NY: Henry Holt and Company, LLC.

31. Somer, E. (1999). Food & Mood. New York, NY: Henry Holt and Company, LLC.

32. Loomis, H.F. (2005). Enzymes, The Key to Health, Volume 1: The Fundamentals. Madison, WI: Grote Publishing

33. Loomis, H.F. (2005). Enzymes, The Key to Health, Volume 1: The Fundamentals. Madison, WI: Grote Publishing

34. Loomis, H.F. (2005). Enzymes, The Key to Health, Volume 1: The Fundamentals. Madison, WI: Grote Publish ing

35. Holford, P. (2004). The New Optimum Nutrition Bible. Berkeley, CA: Crossing Press

36. Morter, M.T. (2000). Fells Official Know-It-All-Guide: Health & Wellness. Hollywood, FL: Frederick Fell Publishers, Inc.

37. Holford, P. (2004). The New Optimum Nutrition Bible. Berkeley, CA: Crossing Press

38. Holford, P. (2004). The New Optimum Nutrition Bible. Berkeley, CA: Crossing Press

39. Brown, S.E., & Trivieri, L. (2006). The Acid-Alkaline Food Guide: A Quick Reference to Foods & Their Effect on

pH Levels. Garden City Park, NY: Square One Publishers

40. Brown, S.E., & Trivieri, L. (2006). The Acid-Alkaline Food Guide: A Quick Reference to Foods & Their Effect on pH Levels. Garden City Park, NY: Square One Publishers

41. Loomis, H.F. (2005). Enzymes, The Key to Health, Volume 1: The Fundamentals. Madison, WI: Grote Publishing

Index

21361503R00049

Made in the USA
Lexington, KY
09 March 2013